Fatigue
Overcome Chronic Fatigue

Discover How To Energize Your Body & Mind So That You Can Bring The Energy & Passion Back Into Your Life

By Ace McCloud
Copyright © 2015

Disclaimer

Table of Contents

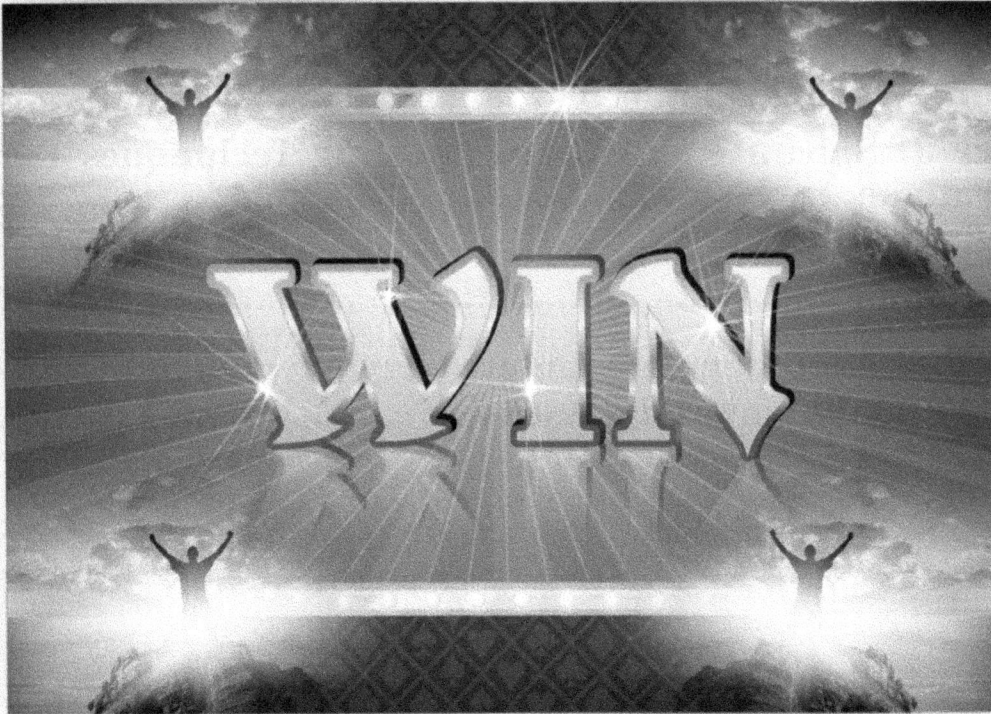

DEDICATED TO THOSE WHO ARE PLAYING THE GAME OF LIFE TO

WIN

KEEP ON PUSHING AND NEVER GIVE UP!

Ace McCloud

Be sure to check out my website for all my Books and Audio books.

www.AcesEbooks.com

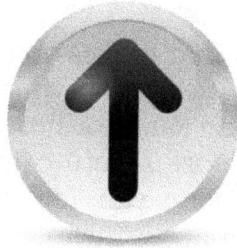

Introduction

I want to thank you and congratulate you for buying this book: "Fatigue: Overcome Chronic Fatigue, Discover How To Energize Your Body & Mind So That You Can Bring The Energy & Passion Back Into Your Life."

Fatigue is like a fog of tiredness that makes you feel like you have no energy or motivation. It is different from drowsiness, which just means that you are tired. Fatigue is a little more intense and can be a little harder to diagnose. It can also be temporary or it could be a more severe condition better known as chronic fatigue syndrome. While everyone can feel tired and worn out, fatigue is definitely something that you do not want to play with. If you do not properly treat fatigue, no matter what level of intensity, it can have some detrimental effects on your life.

Fatigue is notorious for being a major contributing factor in mistakes made by people. Just 17 hours with no sleep can actually make you function the same as if you had a blood alcohol content of 0.05% and spending if you go 24 hours without sleep it can have you functioning as if you had a blood alcohol level of .10%! Fatigue can also cause you to make impaired decisions, ruin your communication skills, reduce your productivity, alter your reaction time, induce forgetfulness and it can increase your risk of getting sick and developing depression. When you are not suffering from fatigue, your productivity levels can soar and you can do amazing things in life. You will be more likely to wake up each day with an energized, refreshed mind—ready to get the day rolling. Your home and work life are more likely to function smoothly and you will likely find yourself happier and more positive.

Fatigue is often a normal reaction to overwork or too much activity and can often be treated with a good night's sleep or some better lifestyle habits. However, some people may discover that those tactics are not working. In those cases, your fatigue may be a bit more severe and will require more care. This book contains proven steps and strategies on how to better understand and recognize fatigue so that you can provide yourself with the best care possible.

In the next couple of pages, you will discover all the best remedies for both chronic and temporary fatigue. You will also discover the most common causes of fatigue, which can serve as a great starting point for anyone who is feeling tired but not sure what may be the underlying cause. There is an entire chapter later in the book dedicated to chronic fatigue syndrome and treatment solutions that you can work toward. You may be surprised at how many different treatment options there are, such as nutritional supplements, physical exercises and mental techniques to name a few. If you suspect that you're only suffering from temporary fatigue, then this book is for you too, as you will discover all the best tactics to safely overcome that slump and come out the other side ready to take on life! Finally, I will take you through a step-by-step process at the end of this book so that you can put your own personal action strategy together that will help you maximize your success potential for conquering the fatigue and tiredness in your life. You won't believe how great you'll be feeling after it's all said and done and you have taken action!

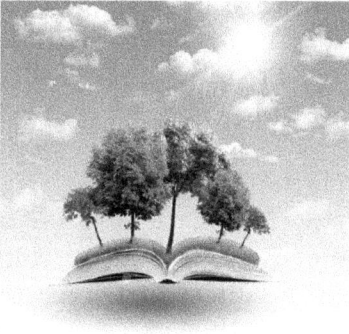

Chapter 1: Why You Get Tired

Fatigue is a symptom of many different conditions and it can also just be a byproduct of how you take care of your body. In this chapter, you will discover some of the most common causes of fatigue. This is a good starting point if you are feeling fatigue but you are not sure where it is coming from. Ask yourself if any of these symptoms apply to you.

Diet is a Top Cause of Fatigue.

The way you manage your diet is often the top cause of many cases of fatigue. Specifically, the more caffeine and sugar you consume, the more likely you are to crash. People commonly think that they can get a nice boost of energy from those sources, but in reality, caffeine and sugar can make you crash even harder. The top peak performers in the world totally avoid caffeine and sugar and are much healthier and productive over the long term because of it.

Fatigue Can Be Caused by Nutritional Deficiencies

Nutritional deficiencies are another one of the top causes of fatigue. Luckily, a nutritional deficiency can often be treated with the right dietary supplement. To find out if you have a deficiency, you can take a self-assessment or undergo a blood test.

Sleeping Habits Play a Big Role in Energy

This one is common knowledge, but your sleeping patterns can play a huge role in how fatigued you may feel. Simply put—the better you can get a good night's rest, the less likely you are to feel fatigued...but if you poorly manage your sleeping habits, you are more likely to feel it.

No Exercise or Too Much Exercise Can Cause Fatigue

Many people commonly believe that exercise can make you tired. The truth is that exercise actually promotes energy, so the more you exercise, the more likely you are to feel energetic. If you don't spend much time exercising, you're more likely to feel fatigued. Additionally, too much exercise can have the opposite effects.

Your Work Environment/Requirements May Be Affecting You...

Research on nurses and fatigue has shown that your work environment can affect how fatigued you are, both mentally and physically. Common factors include long hours and shifts as well as ergonomics (i.e. if you're standing on your feet all day or using poor posture when sitting down).

Toxic Relationships Can Be Draining

Draining relationships can often lead to emotional turmoil and mental distress which can then transform into fatigue.

Alcohol and Drug Abuse Can Lead to Fatigue

Alcohol is a depressant, meaning that it slows down the way your mind functions. Although studies have not found a direct correlation between alcohol use and fatigue, alcohol abuse can often make a case of fatigue worse. Like alcohol, many drugs can slow down your mental functioning and lead to fatigue. For example, people who smoke marijuana often may feel extreme fatigue because it can cause sleepiness.

Fatigue Can Be an Underlying Cause of Hepatitis.

Fatigue is one of the most common symptoms of Hepatitis C and the treatment of Hepatitis C can also cause fatigue.

Fatigue Can Be Caused By Glandular Fever

Glandular Fever, better known as "mono" is an infectious and highly contagious disease that is notorious for causing extreme tiredness in people, along with swollen lymph nodes, sore throat and a high fever.

Fatigue Can Be an Underlying Cause of Anemia

Anemia can be an underlying cause for fatigue and it is especially problematic for women. This can be easily reversed by eating a diet that is full of green vegetables or by taking an iron supplement.

Thyroid Issues May Be Correlated With Fatigue

If your thyroid is over-active or under-active, it can be an underlying cause of fatigue. The best way to confirm this is to undergo a blood test.

Fatigue and Diabetes

Both types of diabetes can make you feel tired out. If you find yourself urinating more than usual and are experiencing blurred vision, your fatigue may be caused by diabetes.

Obesity May Be Linked to Fatigue

Fatigue is sometimes an underlying cause of obesity. Carrying lots of weight around can often be very tiring. Obesity commonly leads to diabetes, which can also cause fatigue.

Depression Can Cause You to Feel Down and Out

If you feel down and out, followed by the loss of interest in doing things you once loved, your fatigue may be an underlying cause of depression. Depression can be a serious issue and you may want to consider enlisting in the help of a good therapist to get back on track.

Fatigue May Be Symptom of Heart Disease

Fatigue is sometimes an underlying cause of heart disease, especially in women. A good way to tell if your fatigue may be generating from heart disease is to evaluate your exercise habits. If you exercise regularly and find it hard to keep up at your regular pace (or if you feel worse when you do exercise) you should consider getting checked out.

Grieving May Lead to Fatigue

Grief, a psychological condition, can be very exhausting. It can often lead to sleeping problems as well as eating problems. Additionally, grief is known to cause mental fatigue.

Fatigue May Be Symptom of Cancer or Side Effect of Cancer Treatment

Cancer (most common in breast cancer). Fatigue is one of the most common side effects of cancer, particularly breast cancer. It can also be caused by treatment such as chemotherapy.

Fatigue May Point to Kidney Disease

Extreme fatigue can be one symptom of kidney disease. This is due to the lack of red blood cells, which carry oxygen.

Chapter 2: Treating Chronic Fatigue Syndrome

What is Chronic Fatigue?

Chronic fatigue syndrome (CFS) is the term that doctors use to describe persistent fatigue, usually caused by a group of other medical conditions. What separates chronic fatigue from normal fatigue is that the symptoms often last for at least six months, are not caused by physical activity and are not cured by sleep. Another factor that makes chronic fatigue syndrome stand out is that there is no single cause, although medical experts believe that it can be caused by brain abnormalities, genetics, immune system problems, viruses, emotional disorders and psychiatric disorders.

Signs and Symptoms of Chronic Fatigue

It is important to educate yourself about the signs and symptoms of chronic fatigue syndrome, as some doctors can misdiagnose it since it is so similar to other illnesses. To demonstrate this, go ahead and type "fatigue" into a search engine and see how many illnesses pop up. Hundreds, right? A skilled doctor can determine chronic fatigue syndrome from other conditions, so it is always important to consult with an expert.

To figure out if you're suffering from chronic fatigue syndrome you should evaluate the nature of your fatigue. Think about a day when you just had a really busy, tiring day at work or a night where you had trouble sleeping and try to remember how you felt. Compare it to the fatigue you are feeling now. If normal rest (both physical and mental) hasn't relieved it and you find yourself functioning well below the level that you usually function at, you may want to consider looking more into chronic fatigue syndrome, especially if the tiredness has lasted for at least six months.

Here are some more symptoms of chronic fatigue syndrome that often follow long-term tiredness:

- Extreme sickness following physical or mental exertion

- Sleeping problems

- Memory and concentration difficulties

- Consistent joint or muscle pain

- Headaches

- Tender lymph nodes

- Sore throat

- Mental fog

- Dizziness

- Fainting

- Balance problems

- Allergies or sensitivity to certain foods, medications, odors, etc

- Sweats and chills

- Depression

- Mood swings

It is important to communicate with your doctor if you are experiencing any of these symptoms. Another important factor to take into consideration is the severity of fatigue. The severity of chronic fatigue syndrome can vary from person to person. Case research has shown that some instances can be mild while others can be as severe as multiple sclerosis. As a rule of thumb, most doctors confirm chronic fatigue syndrome when a patient reports having fatigue for at least six months as well as at least four of the symptoms.

A standard diagnosis for chronic fatigue syndrome requires several steps. First, your doctor will talk to you about your body and ask the right questions so he or she can gain a better understanding of your medical history. Then you will need to have a complete physical examination. Next, your doctor will usually ask you detailed questions about your mental health. After that, your doctor may order some blood tests so that he or she can see what's going on inside of your body. A blood test can often rule out other causes of fatigue that you may be suffering from. If the blood tests show that you may actually *not* have chronic fatigue syndrome, your doctor may order further blood tests. However, if no alternative cause is suspected, he or she will examine your symptoms and the length of time you've been experiencing them to make a diagnosis.

How to Relieve Chronic Fatigue

There is no definitive cure for chronic fatigue syndrome as this book is currently being written. There are so many factors in play and each person is different. Some people may have a complete recovery while others may try all sorts of things with minimal results. Luckily, there are some things that you can do to relieve your symptoms and help make your life more enjoyable. In this section, you will discover some of the best things you can do to help overcome chronic fatigue syndrome and manage it to live a more stress-free and happy life.

- **Exercise Therapy.** Exercise is important for living an overall healthy lifestyle but it can also help patients manage chronic fatigue syndrome, too. Most people choose to exercise on their own but it is different in this case. Since chronic fatigue syndrome is a condition that can weaken one's ability to perform physical activities, this kind of therapy must be handled by an expert who is skilled in CFS cases. Patients usually work with a therapist one-on-one and perform cardio exercises such as swimming or walking. Together, the patient and therapist set goals to gradually increase the intensity of these exercises.

  1. Common exercises for CFS Patients:

     - Walking

     - Water aerobics

     - Swimming

     - Stretching

     - Rowing

- **Cognitive Behavioral Therapy.** Cognitive behavioral therapy is useful for managing the way you mentally deal with fatigue. This type of therapy helps break down the negative emotions that patients associate with CFS to overcome distress. Although CFS is a physical condition and not a mental condition, it can still help to set your mind up for success. Like exercise therapy, cognitive behavioral therapy requires one-on-one work with a professional.

- **Hypnosis Therapy.** Hypnosis is a good way to help yourself relax and build up energy. In a case of chronic fatigue syndrome, hypnosis can help you link your mind and body together to create a sense of vitality and balance. One benefit of hypnosis therapy is that you can do it yourself thanks to recent technology. Hypnosisdownloads.com has some really good packages to choose from. Particularly helpful are the Chronic Fatigue Syndrome package and the 10 Minute Power Nap package.

- **Massage Therapy.** Massage therapy can be very relaxing, both physically and mentally. A massage can be a therapeutic and alternative option to modern medicine. Specifically, a deep tissue massage can be helpful for those with CFS. A massage can help relieve anxiety and help you sleep better at night, thus combatting CFS.

- **Stress Management.** Stress can often make a case of chronic fatigue syndrome go from bad to worse. Although you cannot fully eliminate all stressors from your life, you can learn how to manage them. First, you must learn how to recognize stress. The better you can sense it coming, the better you can deal with it before it takes over. A quick fix easy strategy is to learn how to take deep breaths when you feel yourself getting upset. Ask yourself if you're just being dramatic about something or if it's truly a cause for concern. Sometimes it is easy to just jump into being stressed out over something small. By taking control you put yourself in a much better place to deal with the situation. Stress often stems from fear, so a good idea could be to learn how to overcome your fears.

- **Meditation and Breathing Methods.** Meditating and learning how to pace your breathing can also be very useful alternative options for treating Chronic Fatigue Syndrome. Research shows that these methods can benefit patients because it helps them calm their minds and encourage their bodies to heal. Specifically, meditation can combat stress and anxiety as well as help you get a good night's sleep, all of which you can use to treat CFS.

- **Being Healthy in General.** Whether you suffer from CFS or any other condition, living an overall healthy lifestyle is extremely important for keeping your mind and body in the best condition. However, it can especially help you control and manage CFS. Living a generally healthy lifestyle includes eating a balanced diet, exercising daily, being educated on the healthiest food choices and keeping your mind clear of fog. You should always make it a goal to keep yourself in a healthy condition.

- **Take medication.** Although there is no known absolute cure for all types of Chronic Fatigue Syndrome, there are some that can help to ease the symptoms. Patients commonly take antidepressants to help manage their sleeping patterns. If you are considering medicine as a way to manage CFS, I highly recommend talking to your doctor to pick a medicine that is right for you, as most pharmaceuticals come with some side effects. Most people would agree, however, if you can find ways to all naturally combat your symptoms, then you are generally better off in the long run.

- **Keep a Positive Attitude.** Believe it or not, your attitude can affect how you manage your CFS. People who harness a negative attitude about it are more likely to have a harder time managing it than people who are optimistic and actively striving to combat it's negative effects.

Managing Your Diet With CFS

I mentioned a few moments ago that managing a healthy, balanced diet is important, especially for CFS. Not only can it boost your immune system, strengthen your body and give you more energy, but it may also have a direct effect on how bad CFS affects you. Having to watch your diet for CFS may sound like a pain in the neck, but luckily it is almost identical to watching your diet. This next section will go over some foods that you should incorporate into your diet as well as some foods you should avoid. You will also discover some of the best dietary supplements that you can use.

Foods to avoid:

- Processed foods

- Refined carbohydrates (i.e., sugar or white flour)

- Artificial sweeteners

- Foods with MSG

- Caffeine

- Yeast

Foods to Include:

- Unprocessed or organic foods in general

- Wild-caught fish

- Green vegetables

- Organic eggs

- Organic meat

- Full-fat cheese

- Blueberries

- Blackberries

- Garlic

- Water (up to 8 liters a day)

- Brown rice

- Whole grain oatmeal

- Fruits

- Extra virgin olive oil

- Green tea

As a general rule, you can also experiment with different foods to see how your body reacts and compile your own diet plan.

Dietary Supplements for CFS:

1. Beta-Carotene. Beta-Carotene is an antioxidant that converts itself to Vitamin A and essentially protects your cells from damage and strengthening your immune system. Research shows that short-term use of a beta-carotene supplement can benefit CFS patients.

2. Vitamin C. Vitamin C is another great supplement to help strengthen your immune system and help repair mitochondria. Vitamin C is important for any diet but some research has found that it can also be beneficial for fighting CFS.

3. Zinc. Similar to beta-carotene and vitamin c, zinc is also useful for boosting your immune system and may be helpful for CFS.

4. Sodium. While it is important to watch your sodium intake in a regular diet, some research has shown that a sodium deficiency may have an indirect impact on patients with CFS. This may be something that you might talk to your doctor about investigating.

5. Omega-3 Fatty Acids. Omega-3 fatty acids are good antioxidants and they can also contribute to yeast overgrowth management, which may help combat some of the symptoms of CFS.

6. Caprylic Acid. This supplement is useful for controlling yeast overgrowth as well, especially if you have an acidic body.

7. B Vitamins. B vitamins help your nervous system function and help oxygen flow well in your body. Most importantly, a vitamin b complex can help your body generate energy for its cells.

8. Coenzyme Q10. Coenzyme Q10 is a strong antioxidant that promotes energy throughout your body. It also can help boost the health of your heart.

9. Adrenal Extracts. Adrenal extracts are chemically processed supplements taken from animal adrenal glands that can help those who are suffering from fatigue and low adrenal function. Some people believe that the adrenal extracts from an animal's gland can help their own adrenal glands function although every person's body reacts differently. There are many types of adrenal extracts to choose from but the top two that I have seen are Adrenal Support and Adrenal Edge.

All Natural Approaches to Treating CFS

- Fenugreek. Fenugreek is a herbal supplement that helps fend off depression, stress and fatigue, all of which are major symptoms of CFS.

- Ghee. Ghee is an all-natural supplement that can strengthen your immune system and help you become more energetic as well as boost your memory function, which is always a plus.

- Cinnamon. Cinnamon, which you can find in almost any spice section at the grocery store, is great for treating CFS because it is another really awesome immune system strengthener.

- Ginseng. Research in Asia has showed that ginseng effectively helped those who were suffering from chronic fatigue.

Lifestyle Habits for Treating CFS

1. Form Good Sleeping Habits. This may be hard at first but it can be a very crucial step in treating CFS. There is actually a lot more to forming good sleeping habits than many people think. First and foremost, you should sleep in an area that is completely dark and free from noise or other distractions that could disturb you. Also, make sure that your pillow is fairly new and comfortable. An old pillow can become flat and fail to provide support. You should also check the quality of your bed—sometimes those old spring mattresses just don't cut the job. An investment into a more modern, more comfortable bed may be a wise investment. The recommended amount of sleep for an adult is between 6 and 8 hours a night.

2. Incorporate Basic Stretches. While you should consult with an expert when it comes to actual exercises, it can be safe to do some stretching on your own. This can help you stay active and flexible as well as keep your joints moving. All you need to do is set aside 10 minutes for stretching each day. Just do basic stretches, such as reaching your hands toward the sky and touching your toes, it doesn't have to be anything fancy. Sit-ups and push-ups are okay too as long as you don't over-exert yourself.

3. Schedule Regular Doctor Visits. Since CFS is such a complex condition, it is very important to work closely with your doctor to make sure that you are making the right decisions and taking the right medicines/supplements. Your doctor can ultimately give you the best advice regarding your body, as he or she will know your complete medical history and will be able to guide you that way. This is also important because the more time you spend at the doctor's, the more likely you are to be in overall good health. Additionally, your doctor will be able to monitor your progress as well as help you manage your stress levels.

4. Be Proud of Who You Are. One common mistake that CFS patients make is that they compare themselves to each other and that can sometimes get pretty discouraging. The key is to keep a good attitude about your condition and be proud of who you are. Every CFS patient responds differently to medicines, diets, supplements and treatment programs. Try to focus more on your success rather than of your downfalls.

5. Make Friends with Others Who Suffer From CFS. It is possible to feel alone when you have CFS. You might feel like you're the only one who understands what you're going through. If you can, try to make some friends with others who are in the same boat as you. Having friends who understand what you're going through can be very comforting and supportive and it may actually inspire you to stay positive throughout your journey.

Chapter 3: Curing Temporary Fatigue

Temporary fatigue is common in people who are often overworked, overtired or a combination of both. You have probably experienced temporary fatigue at some point in your life. If so, then you know that it is easy to find the root cause of it and there are some easy cures. Determining whether you are suffering from temporary fatigue is pretty easy. The symptoms usually include feelings of weakness, exhaustion, lack of energy/motivation, having a hard time concentrating and/or having a hard time finishing your job(s).

Temporary fatigue can be very frustrating, especially to a person with a busy life, so this chapter is going to go over everything you can do to prevent or cure it.

As you know, the most common causes of temporary fatigue stem out of lifestyle habits. These habits commonly include excessive alcohol use, excessive caffeine use, too much physical activity, a lack of physical activity, over-the-counter medications (usually cough syrups), poor sleeping habits and/or unhealthy dietary habits. There are a few psychological factors that can also contribute to fatigue, including anxiety, depression, grief and stress. Certain medical issues can cause fatigue too. This commonly includes anemia, COPD, heart disease, thyroid disorders, obesity and diabetes.

Fast, Easy and All Natural Cures for Temporary Fatigue

- Add two drops of peppermint oil to a handkerchief and place it on your nose while breathing deeply. Alternatively, you can add a few drops of peppermint to your bathwater for a nice, relaxing bath before bed.

- Lay down with your feet elevated. Some believe that you can fight fatigue by encouraging blood flow to your head.

- Make sure you eat a full, balanced breakfast. Breakfast is the most important meal of the day and it can set the stage for your body until later in the night. A healthy breakfast generally means a more energetic day and you can unwind when you're getting ready for bed. I like to start off the day by first drinking a huge cup of water, then 15 minutes later drinking a large cup of wheat grass powder mixed in water, doing a good stretching routine, then having a smoothie consisting of a banana and spinach or baby spinach. I will then go on a run/walk, come back and have another smaller energy meal, which can be something like almonds or oatmeal. Be sure to try eating more frequent but smaller meals throughout the day, this can seriously help out the majority of people!

- Dice an unpeeled tomato and soak the pieces in water while you sleep. In the morning, drink the water for a nice potassium boost. Experts in the "all-natural" field believe that your body can benefit from potassium in the morning, especially for those who have a deficiency.

- Eat as much spinach as you can (it's not that bad!). Spinach is another source of potassium and it's a leafy green, which can be good for beating fatigue and being healthy overall.

- Stay hydrated. Experts recommend drinking at least eight glasses of water each day. Dehydration can easily tire you out.

- Exercise for at least thirty minutes a day. Focus on aerobics. Not only can this help fend off fatigue but it can also keep you fit and help you sleep better at night.

- Additionally, take a little stroll during the day if you're feeling sluggish. This can wake you up a little and help you stay more alert.

- Implement good sleeping habits into your daily routine. One mistake that many people make is that they don't have a set sleeping schedule. This can be challenging for those who work a job with changing hours but with a little strategy, you can come up with a plan. You should try to get up and go to sleep at the same time every night. Even if you have to wake up at 5am on the weekdays, keep getting up at that time even on the weekends. This will help your body get on a set sleep schedule and it will be easier to sleep at night.

- Don't take long naps. Long naps can be tempting but they can actually make you more tired. Instead, just take short naps. Set a timer if you have too.

If you follow these steps/tips, you should easily be able to cure your fatigue. If your symptoms are persistent, you may want to talk to your doctor about looking into whether you have chronic fatigue syndrome. Also, you should try to quit smoking if you have a tendency to light up.

Useful Items to Help Prevent Fatigue

In additional to all-natural cures, there are some investments that you can make to help improve the quality of your daily life and prevent fatigue. This section will help you get some ideas on things that you can incorporate into your life to stop getting overtired.

- **Anti-Fatigue Mats.** If you have a job that requires you to stand on your feet all day in a stationary position (or if you do anything that requires you to be on your feet in a standing position for long periods of time), you can invest in <u>an anti-fatigue mat</u>. These mats are designed to give your body better support.

- **Anti-Fatigue Insoles.** Alternatively, you could opt to put <u>anti-fatigue insoles</u> in your shoes. This is a good idea if you're on your feet all day but moving around a lot.

- **Sleep Mask and Ear Plugs.** If you're having trouble sleeping at night, you can invest in a <u>sleep mask and pair of ear plugs</u>. Sometimes you will have to eliminate distractions to get a better night's sleep.

Chapter 4: Spiritual and Brain Boosting Techniques that Fight Fatigue

In addition to fighting fatigue with supplements or exercise, there are some spiritual/brain-boosting techniques that you can also try out. In this chapter, you will discover some of the best spiritual and mental techniques to beat physical/mental fatigue. I think you will find these methods very relaxing and beneficial to your life.

Spiritual Techniques:

- **Meditation.** Meditating can be helpful in fighting fatigue because it can help prevent anxiety and stress, two symptoms of fatigue. Research also shows that it can help reduce insomnia. Learning how to meditate can be fairly simple and you can practice it almost anywhere. Sit in a quiet area in a comfortable position, keeping your back straight. Slightly close your eyes and begin to focus on your breathing, concentrating on how it works. You may be tempted to start focusing on your thoughts but, every time that happens, refocus on your breathing. This may take a little practice but it is a great way to calm your mind and induce relaxation.

- **The Emotional Freedom Technique.** This technique, sometimes referred to as "tapping," is used to eliminate any emotional problems that a person may be suffering from to lessen the effects of a physical ailment. It is based off ancient Chinese beliefs that energy circuits in your body can be "tapped" to alter your physical/emotional health. To see this technique in action, watch this video: Emotional Freedom Technique EFT ho'oponopono by Alexander Wilson.

- **The Wisdom-Lotus Qigong Technique.** This technique, also derived from the ancient Chinese, is a visualization method that can help you achieve a clear mind. To perform this technique, sit somewhere quiet (indoors or outdoors is fine). Start by imagining the sun moving towards you from the sky, gradually warming you up. Then visualize it shrinking into a small ball that glows inside your stomach. Next, picture a giant lotus approaching you. Sit on the lotus and let the sun inside of you connect with its leaves—picture this for about three minutes. Again, picture the lotus shrinking and moving inside of you like the sun. After that, picture the lotus moving clockwise and counterclockwise a few times, making the circular movements bigger and smaller respectively. Focus on this image for another three minutes and then you're done.

- **Transcendental Meditation.** This type of meditation stems from India and was introduced by Maharashi Mahesh. To perform transcendental meditation, simply sit in a comfortable position in a comfortable space and close your eyes. Pick a mantra (How to Choose Your Mantra and Four

Additional Tips on YouTube by drnespor can help in choosing) and silently repeat it to yourself. Experts believe that doing this can help you achieve a state of stability, stillness and perfect consciousness.

- **Reflective Meditation.** Reflective meditation is the practice of disciplined thinking, in which you focus your thoughts on a specific question or set of questions. This can help you control your mind better and stop it from zoning off, which can prevent anxiety. Many people choose to focus on the question, "What is the true purpose of my life?", although you can reflect on anything. Here is some Reflective Piano Music For Relaxing, Meditation and Contemplation by PureInstrumentals on YouTube.

- **Kundalini.** Kundalini is a type of meditation in which you become more aware of the energy that is rising over you. When a person practices this type of meditation, he or she focuses on their breathing so that it helps the energy rise up.

- **Qi Gong.** Qi Gong is a Taoist-based type of meditation that also focuses on the flow of energy throughout your body. The practice of Qi Gong allows energy to circulate throughout your organs as you focus on three major points: one located two inches below your belly button, one located in the center of your chest and the other in the center of your forehead. Here is some Qi Gong Music Sounds: Relaxing Tai Chi Music and QiGong Meditation Music by BuddhaTribe on YouTube.

Brain Boosting/Mental Techniques:

If you are fatigued. it can negatively affect your brain as well as your body. Specifically, it can impact your ability to pay attention, think clearly and recall things in your memory. Sleep deprivation itself can also have similar impacts on your brain. Here are some great brain boosting techniques to fight fatigue and ensure mental clarity:

- **Time your meals to occur before big events.** For example, if you're preparing to take a huge exam, eat an hour or so beforehand so the nutrients can make their way to your brain and help you focus better. If you eat right before a big event it can actually perform worse.

- **Clear your brain of worrying by practicing breathing exercises and stress management techniques.** You can also try to keep your life more organized by keeping goal trackers and to-do lists, which can take some weight off your memory.

  o **Breathing Exercise #1:**

    1. Place one hand on your chest and the other on your belly.

2. Sigh and let your upper body relax as you breathe out.

3. Close your mouth and don't do anything for a few seconds.

4. Without opening your mouth, slowly inhale and push your belly out at the same time.

5. Pause for as long as you need.

6. Breathe out through your mouth while pulling your belly back in.

7. Rest again and then repeat steps 2 through 6.

- **Breathing Exercise #2:**

  1. Inhale and push out your belly while counting to five.

  2. Exhale and pull in your belly while counting to five.

  3. Do this until you've taken six complete breaths.

  4. This method helps your heart get in sync with the endorphins in your brain, which can help you feel good.

- **Breathing Exercise #3:**

  1. Start out by breathing like you tried in exercise #1 or exercise #2.

  2. Two minutes into your breathing, start focusing on your heart. A good way to do this is to think about someone who you truly love. Think about how much this person means to you and try to visualize the love you feel for him or her flowing through your heart.

  3. Next, slowly picture the image of that person disappearing but hold on to the feelings that you're feeling.

  4. Experts believe that this type of breathing can help your overall well-being.

- Reward yourself for hard work. Don't try to be serious all the time or you risk mental burnout which can lead to mental fatigue. Be sure to take some leisurely time to yourself.

- Try to simplify your life in any way possible. For example, you can minimize distractions (cell phones, TV, radio, etc.) when you're focusing on a really important task.

- Don't be afraid to step outside and get some fresh air. This is especially important if you sit in front of a computer or an indoor job all day. Some people find nature to be very relaxing.

- Try out a brain dumping exercise. Brain dumping is when you freely write down your thoughts and anything else that comes to your mind for a good 15 minutes. You can handwrite it or type it out on your computer. Some people find this useful for clearing all the thoughts in your head while you're still awake.

Chapter 5: How To Conquer Your Fatigue Once and For All

Putting everything that you've learned so far together is the most important step for success. Whether you are suffering from chronic fatigue syndrome or temporary fatigue, I will help you put together an action plan in this last chapter that you can use for a lifetime, or until you have fully learned to manage/treat your condition. I truly hope this action plan will be able to help you empower yourself and live every day with as much energy as possible.

Step 1) Try to determine what type of fatigue you have—chronic or temporary. Knowing which type you are suffering from can be beneficial when you begin planning. If you're really not sure which type you are dealing with, you can ask your doctor.

Step 2) Set a goal to conquer your fatigue. You may be tempted to just go into this without literally stating your goal, but doing that can help increase your chances of being successful by over 50%. Additionally, if you visualize your goal(s), you are three times more likely to be successful. I recommend setting a long-term goal to ultimately overcome fatigue and then setting 3-5 short-term goals to help get you there.

Here is a great example of how you can do this:

Long-Term Goal: I will easily overcome my temporary fatigue (or manage my chronic fatigue).

Say this goal out loud and even write it down. I like to write my goals down on sticky notes and hang them by my computer to remind me, but you can write them anywhere you look all the time. Next, start planning out your short-term goals. For this example, we will pretend that you're going to overcome temporary fatigue.

Short-Term Goal #1: I will easily start regulating my sleeping patterns.

You can break this goal down even more by narrowing in on the specifics—will you invest in new pillows? Will you make your sleeping area even darker? Will you start going to bed and waking up at the same time every day?

Short-Term Goal #2: I will easily change my diet to make myself feel better.

You can also break this goal down as well by deciding what you want to add and take away from your diet to become more energized. I recommended including this as one of your short-term goals no matter what your situation is because eating right can make you feel great overall. I highly recommend my book: Ultimate Energy if you would like even more ideas how to become more energized in your life!

Short-Term Goal #3: I will easily add more exercise to my life.

I think a lot of people shy away from the exercise part because they think they have to dedicate a great deal of time to it. Even if you just gradually start exercising, you'll be okay. You may even find that you enjoy exercising and you will want to start doing it more eventually. Depending on your home and work situation, you can either go to the gym and really dedicate yourself to exercising or just do something as simple as take a short walk on your down time. Walking is incredibly beneficial and very healthful for just about everyone!

Notice that I only listed 3 short-term goals. You should aim to set at least 3 to 5 short-term goals for every long-term goal that you set so you don't overload yourself.

Step 3) Now that you know how to set goals to combat fatigue, the next step is to customize these goals to your life. Since no two people are alike and I cannot speak for everyone, there is no "one size fits all" action plan that I can write here. What I can do is encourage you to brainstorm the top 25 things that you can do to help fight your fatigue. For this exercise, I want you to really think about your life, your home environment, your work environment and your capabilities. Go into this exercise with an open mind and don't hold anything back—nobody will see this plan but you if that's how you want it to be.

Here are some more ideas to consider:

- Is there any way you can arrange your hours at work to be more consistent?

- Can you find a better way to delegate some of your tasks so all the heat is not on you?

- Is your whole family willing to get on a consistent sleep pattern?

- What can you and your partner do if you both have different sleep patterns?

- Do you have any consistent down time during the day to spend taking naps?

- How much are you willing to work exercise into your lifestyle?

- Do you get an annual check up to make sure that you're not developing any conditions that cause fatigue?

o   Are you willing to wean yourself off caffeine for long term benefit?

o   Are you willing to mentally focus on beating the fatigue in your life?

o   What are your favorite ways to relax?

Go ahead and do your brainstorming. I will see you at Step 4.

Step 4) If you've made it to this step, then you have your 25 customized ideas on how you can combat the fatigue that is driving you down. Now that your brain is really warmed up, I want you to analyze that list and pick out the top 5 options that you think are most **practical** and **realistic**. I am sure that thinking of 25 ideas caused you to rack your brain a little and possibly throw out some ideas that may sound a bit farfetched or stretched. For example, you may have suggested that your entire family go to sleep and get up at the same time—but if you have one child in elementary school, one in high school and your partner works the overnight shift while you work the morning shift—that is probably not going to work out.

Step 5) The last and final step is to ensure that you are implementing these goals and ideas into your life. I know from experience that using a calendar tool helps me stay organized and it helps me achieve all of my daily goals. You can use a traditional calendar or a digital one. I always plan out my weeks one week ahead of time and I always check off my tasks as I complete them to make sure I've covered them all.

Conclusion

Fatigue can be tiring, demoralizing and depressing, but this book should give you many powerful tools that you can immediately put into place in order to help you overcome or manage fatigue. Be sure to take action immediately while you are feeling motivated and implement your new favorite strategies into your life!

The next step is to figure out what will work best for you. Hopefully you were able to get a good idea about what's causing you're fatigue. Once you have found the root cause or have a pretty good idea of it, then it is up to you to determine how you want to go about treating/managing it. My recommendation would be to reevaluate your life and pick out everything that would be easy to change. Make those changes into habits, and then be sure to use visualization and motivation techniques to make sure your goals are accomplished! Be sure to follow the action plan you created in chapter 5, and remember to never give up! Hopefully sooner, rather than later, you will discover exactly what you need to do in order to live an energy filled and happy life!

Finally, if you discovered at least one thing that has helped you or that you think would be beneficial to someone else, be sure to take a few seconds to easily post a quick positive review. As an author, your positive feedback is desperately needed. Your highly valuable five star reviews are like a river of golden joy flowing through a sunny forest of mighty trees and beautiful flowers! *To do your good deed in making the world a better place by helping others with your valuable insight, just leave a nice review.*

Thanks and Best of Luck

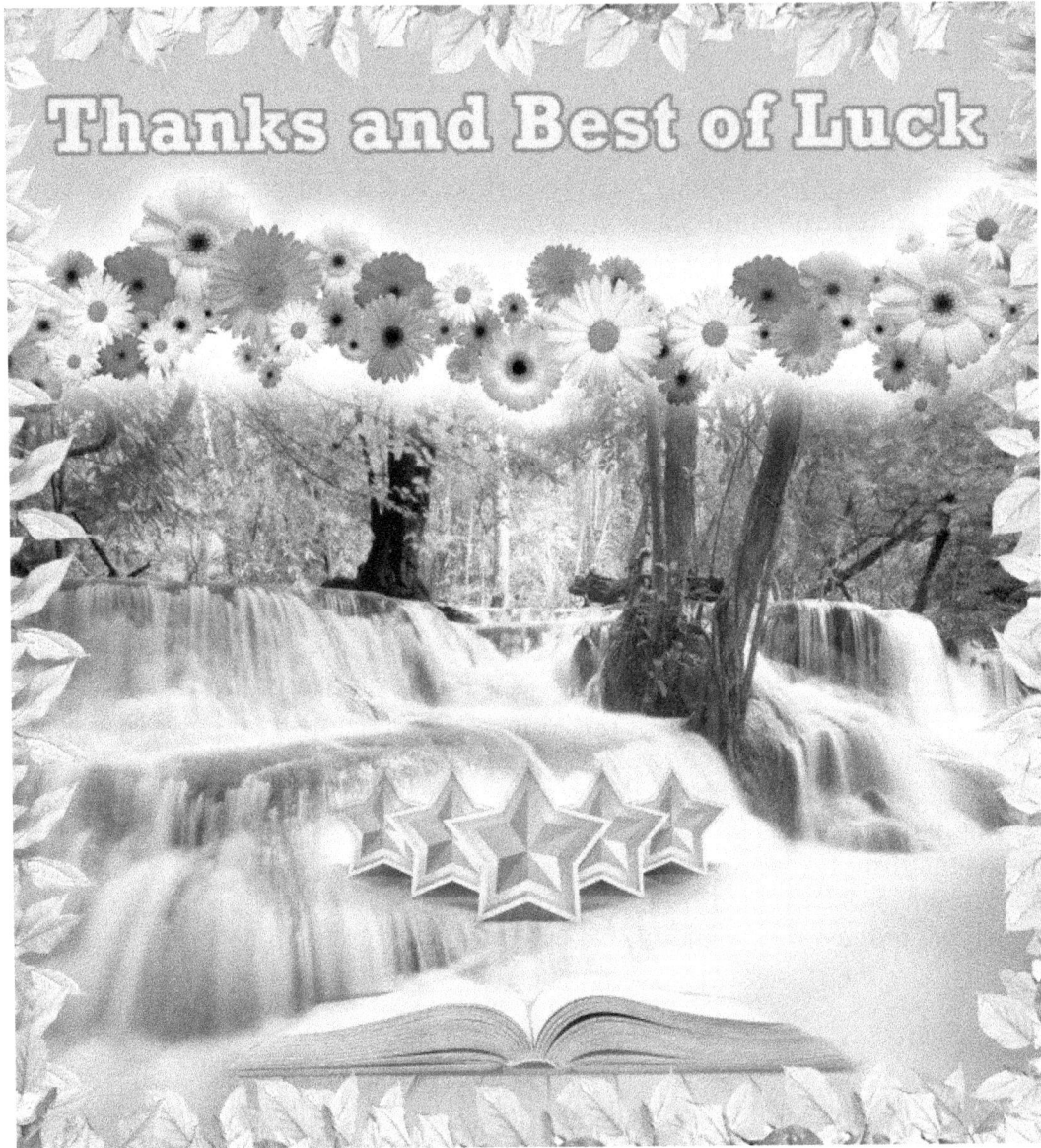

My Other Books and Audio Books
www.AcesEbooks.com

Health Books

ULTIMATE HEALTH SECRETS

HEALTH

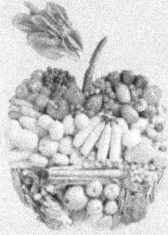

Strategies For Dieting, Eating Healthy, Exercising,
Losing Weight, The Mediterranean Diet,
Strength Training, And All About Vitamins,
Minerals, And Supplements

Ace McCloud

ENERGY
ULTIMATE ENERGY

Discover How To Increase
Your Energy Levels
Using The Best All Natural
Foods, Supplements
And Strategies For A Life
Full Of Abundant Energy

Ace McCloud

RECIPE BOOK

The Best Food Recipes
That Are Delicious, Healthy,
Great For Energy And Easy To Make

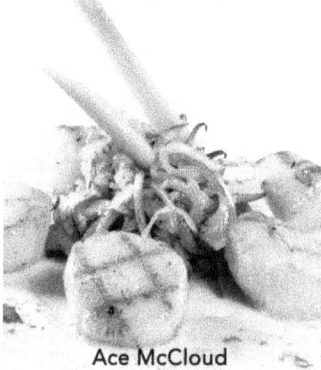

Ace McCloud

MASSAGE THERAPY

TRIGGER POINT THERAPY
ACUPRESSURE THERAPY
Learn The Best Techniques For
Optimum Pain Relief And Relaxation

Ace McCloud

LOSE WEIGHT

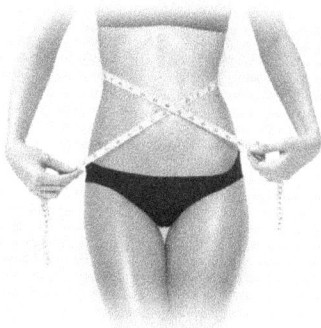

THE TOP 100 BEST WAYS
TO LOSE WEIGHT QUICKLY AND HEALTHILY

Ace McCloud

FATIGUE
OVERCOME CHRONIC FATIGUE

Discover How To Energize
Your Body & Mind So
That You Can Bring
The Energy & Passion
Back Into Your Life

Ace McCloud

Peak Performance Books

SUCCESS
SUCCESS STRATEGIES
THE TOP 100 BEST WAYS TO BE SUCCESSFUL

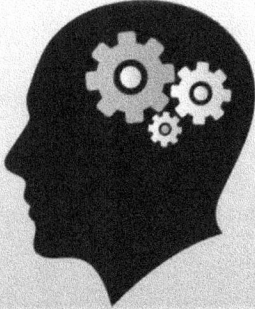

Ace McCloud

Ace McCloud

HABIT

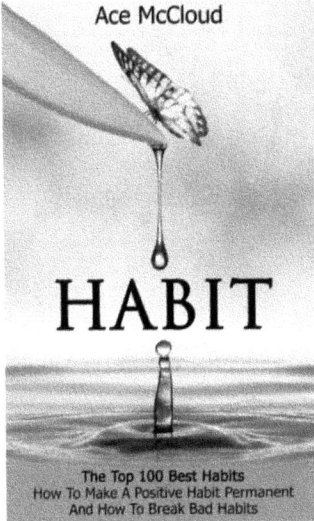

The Top 100 Best Habits
How To Make A Positive Habit Permanent
And How To Break Bad Habits

MOTIVATION
MASTER THE POWER OF MOTIVATION
TO PROPEL YOURSELF TO SUCCESS

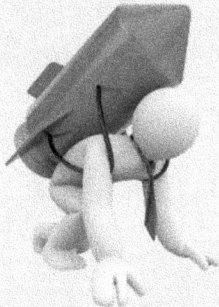

Ace McCloud

ATTITUDE
Discover The True Power Of
A Positive Attitude

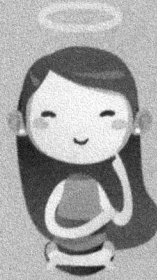

Ace McCloud

SELF DISCIPLINE
Unleash The Power Of Self Discipline, Influence And Willpower In Your Life To Achieve Anything
Ace McCloud

Competitive Strategies
WINNING STRATEGIES
The Top 100 Best Strategies For Peak Performance During Competitions
Ace McCloud

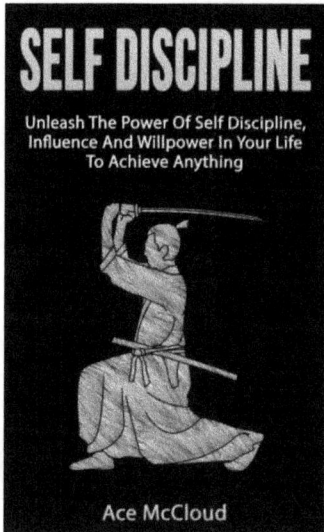

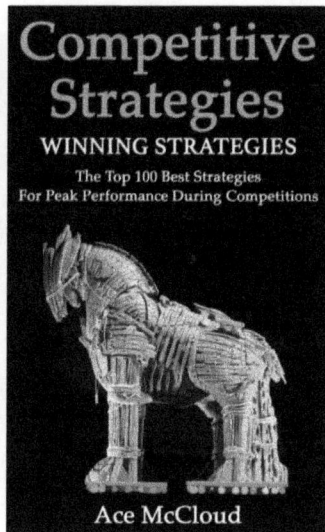

Be sure to check out my audio books as well!

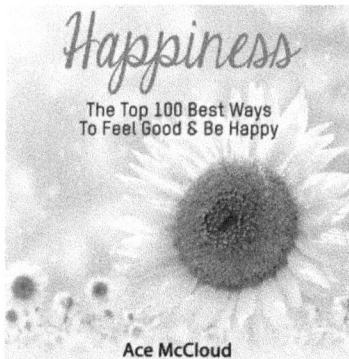

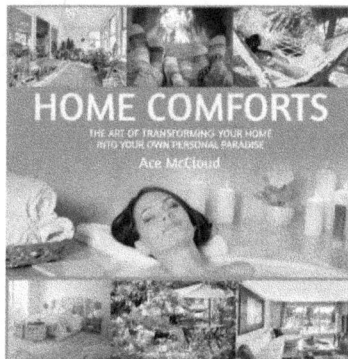

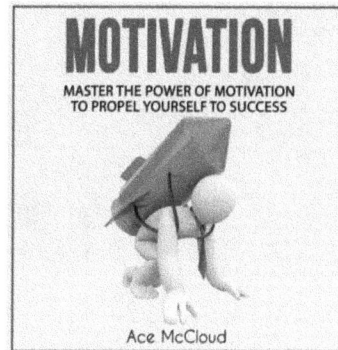

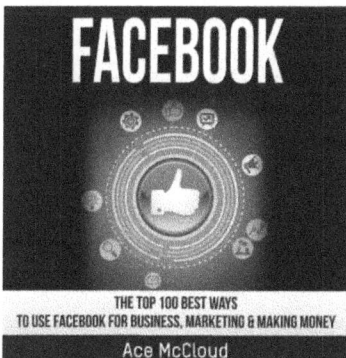

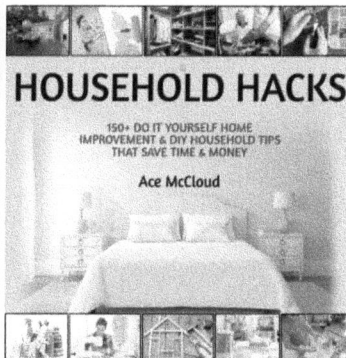

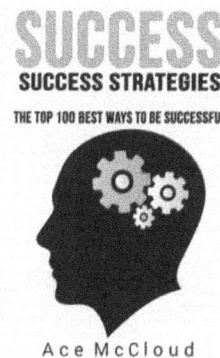

Happiness
The Top 100 Best Ways To Feel Good & Be Happy
Ace McCloud

HOME COMFORTS
THE ART OF TRANSFORMING YOUR HOME INTO YOUR OWN PERSONAL PARADISE
Ace McCloud

MOTIVATION
MASTER THE POWER OF MOTIVATION TO PROPEL YOURSELF TO SUCCESS
Ace McCloud

FACEBOOK
THE TOP 100 BEST WAYS TO USE FACEBOOK FOR BUSINESS, MARKETING & MAKING MONEY
Ace McCloud

HOUSEHOLD HACKS
150+ DO IT YOURSELF HOME IMPROVEMENT & DIY HOUSEHOLD TIPS THAT SAVE TIME & MONEY
Ace McCloud

SUCCESS
SUCCESS STRATEGIES
THE TOP 100 BEST WAYS TO BE SUCCESSFUL
Ace McCloud

Check out my website at: **www.AcesEbooks.com** for a complete list of all of my books and high quality audio books. I enjoy bringing you the best knowledge in the world and wish you the best in using this information to make your journey through life better and more enjoyable! **Best of luck to you!**

www.ingramcontent.com/pod-product-compliance
Lightning Source LLC
Chambersburg PA
CBHW080632030426
42336CB00018B/3175